Dr Bodo Koehler, MD

MANUAL of the UNITED life supporting MEDICINE

Reproduction or duplication, in whole or in part,
requires the written consent of the author.

2st edition 2020

Production and publishing:
BoD-Books on Demand, Norderstedt

ISBN 9-783734-76306-9

The work including all its parts is protected by copyright. Any use outside the narrow limits of copyright law without the consent of the author is inadmissible and punishable. This applies in particular to reproductions, microfilming and the transfer to electronic data carriers.

All rights reserved by the author Bodo Koehler, MD

Foreword

After the publication of the more then 500-pages "Textbook of the UNITED life supporting MEDICINE", the need for a short version for daily practice emerged. In this manual, therefore, the main cornerstones are summarized again. However, it cannot replace all the details of the textbook and the extensive explanations. For the start into the future of ***one united*** medicine, a comprehensive and repeated study of the fundamentals is inevitable.

The most important thing is the extension of the personal worldview. For it depends entirely on which spectacles through which we see reality and what becomes reality for us. The same applies to the consideration of illnesses and the evaluation of our patients seeking help. We can do much more for them and treat them much more successfully once we understand what and at what level the problems actually occurred. This allows the crucial ***causal*** access.

Some keywords will repeat more often because they are the cornerstones by which we base our considerations:
Coherence, ***bipolar regulation*** and ***reciprocity*** (affects all functional systems), ***information*** (the spiritual aspect of matter) as well as ***charge carriers*** (in particular electrons and protons are responsible for the energetic aspect).

A core sentence represents the foundation upon which we should be guided: ***Spirit creates and controls matter***. Our emotionally generated intentions determine our actions and thus all bodily functions. It is they who can maintain health or cause disease through our motivation. The most important thing is to strictly adhere to the basic law of ***giving and giving back***.

Also with this book my beloved wife Helga provided for corrections and the necessary fine tuning, for which I am very grateful to her.

I wish you every success with the future of medicine!

The Author   spring 2020

Content

Introduction
Matter	6
Energy	6
Information	7
Spirit	7
Quantum physics	8
Interactions	8
Life	10
Health	10
UNITED life supporting MEDICIN ULM	11
The scientific basis	13
Psycho regulation, question of sense, personal worldview	13
The 3 + 1 law a.t. W. Pauli and the bipolar regulation	13
The categorical ORDER SYSTEM	15
The uniform REFERENCE SYSTEM	16

Pathogenesis
Excessive demand	20
Chronic inflammation	21
Toxic loads	21
Deficiency states versus overloading	22
Psycho regulation	22
Reciprocity	24

Diagnostics
Case history	28
Questionnaire for the case history	29
Personality assessment	30
Bioenergetics testing	31
Imaging procedures	32
Laboratory analyses	33
Special features and standard values	33
Example of a laboratory order	36

Therapy

Reciprocal treatment — 37
Mother and father principle — 38
Coherence therapy CHT — 41
Balancing therapy with Equalizer EQ 103 — 43
Key points for LSM therapy — 45

Lifestyle

Sense of life, life task — 46
Nutrition — 47
Rough division of food & beverages — 48
Movement — 54
Sleep — 55
Epilogue — 55

List of Figures 1 — 57

Literature — 60

Attachment

4 aspects of body organization — 62
Application of the categorical classification system — 66
Load capacity of the organism — 69
Consequences — 70

List of Figures 2 — 72

Introduction

In summary, the features of the new science paradigm are presented here. These compressed contents should be completely internalized, as they form the basis for all thinking and acting in personal life – now and in the future. They shape your own worldview. Big changes can only be implemented from a new perspective. This is especially true for medicine.

MATTER consists only of the one-billionth part of mass whose ordered structure is given by *information*. The predominant part is *interaction quanta*. These can either be considered as points or particles (virtual and real photons) in the 3rd dimension or as waves in the 4th dimension (function of time). These create fields. Both states are in a reciprocal relation to each other (1 / x) and are constantly transforming into each other. That is, there is no wave-particle dualism (either-or), but one *polarity* – as-well-as. Both states exist side by side. The material *shapes* are maintained by electrical tensions (potentials). Information-bearing *electrons* play the main role here. These force effects are an expression of the unlimited vacuum energy (zero-point energy).

ENERGY itself is not measurable. It is the counter pol of *information* and like this an inherent property of the mind (unified field). It is only recognizable by its power effects. Their carriers are the photons (quantum of light), which, as so-called QuBits, contain an enormous amount of energy and information at the same time, well over 10^{30} Bits. Therefore, only 1 photon is required to trigger 1 trillion (10^9) chemical reactions. This benefits cell metabolism. The necessary information comes only partially from the DNA. Our genome is way too small for that. The larger part comes from the natural environment fields we are constantly resonating with, both through food and directly. In the middle of nature we succeed best; it's getting harder in big cities and can be a problem. Frequent walks in the sunshine in the countryside, especially in the forest, sustainably promote good health.

INFORMATION is fundamentally attributable to the spirit and belongs to the 7th and 8th dimension according to the physics-chemist Burkhard Heim. But it can only take effect if it is given *meaning*. This is an act of consciousness and therefore reserved for living systems. The quantum physicist Thomas Goernitz distinguishes *meaningful, material-structuring* and *energy-donating information*. This is in a polar relationship to the energy. It cannot take effect without a small amount of energy for its transmission. Nor can energy take effect without giving appropriate information. The information is encoded in the spin.

SPIRIT can be scientifically described also as a *unified field* (of all laws of nature). There are other terms such as zero point fields, vacuum field, potential field and others. These fields contain an inexhaustible potential of *possibilities* that can be retrieved via emotions. Every idea comes from there. It can be charged with emotions and then becomes information.

Spirit rests in itself, but at the same time shows a high dynamic (fluctuations of virtual fields). By contacting the resting mind – e.g. in a meditation – an expansion of consciousness can be effected and necessary healing information can be called up. This was proven by means of nuclear spin recordings.

QUANTUM MECHANICS is the doctrine of the whole, of the unity from which everything emerges and in which everything is connected with everything. It deals with the *interactions* that take place *between* the material facts, whereby the facts themselves only have the role of extras, for which classical physics is responsible. Since material facts and thus mass particles make up only a tiny fraction of reality, quantum mechanics is valid for all areas, not just for quanta.

It is able to scientifically grasp and experimentally prove all relationships and the resulting possibilities (interactions). In particular, it is able to represent *life processes* based on information transmissions through real photons. As *virtual* photons, they are also responsible for all power effects. According to the statements of important quantum physicists, there is a higher intelligence behind these encompassing properties of *light*.

INTERACTIONS

All material forms are subject to a high dynamics of creation and dissolution. They are subject to equally high dynamics of *interactions* with each other. In this way everything is interwoven with everything and inseparably connected. When describing a condition, e.g. a source of illness, then it seems stable to us. In reality, however, it is *a process that has been disturbed in its adaptability*. If we approach a patient from this point of view, something non-material is in the foreground, namely the informative-energetic aspect, and that is what matters.

We are continuously shaped by all the influences we are exposed to, right through to advertising. Over time, an enormous potential of *information waste* accumulates, which we can dispose of only partially in the sleep over dreams. This not only increases the disease readiness, but also creates problems for the treatment. The responsiveness for informative therapies, which includes homeopathy, but also the Living Systems Information Therapy LSIT, is decreasing.

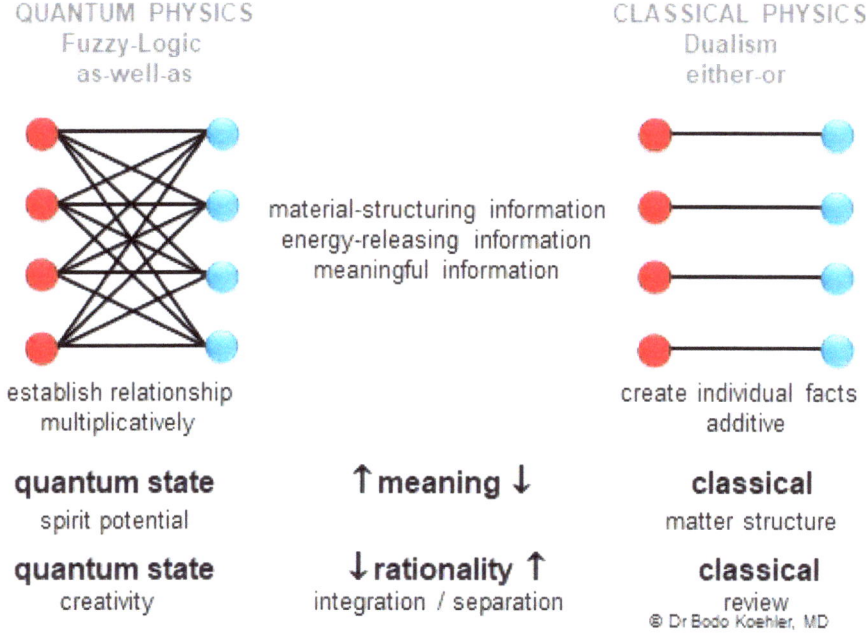

Fig.1: Quantum physics describes interactions (Th. Goernitz)

For health maintenance we need a high proportion of natural signals, which we get, for example during walking in the forest from the living nature and directly from the sun. If this input is missing, this is at the expense of the structure. An important part is also the communication with other people. The more high-quality conversations we have, the more our mind is stimulated, and thus the creative potential, which is also responsible for renewal and regeneration. The counterexample we see in old people who break down very quickly after moving to the retirement home.

LIFE is a rhythmic sequence of *complex networked processes* that are psychically controlled and based on the all-encompassing knowledge of the structure-building, universal spirit. All life processes are subject to a bipolar (four-pole) control and thus fulfil the 3 + 1 law according to Wolfgang Pauli. The necessary material structures are quickly dissolved and re-formed, just as the whole universe is subject to constant change. Consistent is only the divine plan.

HEALTH depends on 4 aspects that should be lived out individually for constitutional reasons:
- Lifestyle and meaningful task
- adapted biologically high-quality diet
- adequate movement, without overloading
- restful sleep between 7 and 9 hours

Who consistently adheres to all points, has the best chances, not to get seriously ill. These are the crucial aspects that every human being can contribute to. This ensures that the organism can maintain its ability to adapt quickly to changing environmental conditions to ensure dynamic balance (homeo-dynamics). For this, a labile regulatory capacity is required, which is made possible by the cell metabolism. Together with the regulation of the acids-base balance, this results in the *cell-milieu system*. It is the smallest, autonomously functioning unit.

The basic regulation of the **cell metabolism** occurs purely via so-called *electron*-donor-acceptor reactions, i.e. the uptake and release of electrons. The **pH value** is controlled by *protons*. Both charge carriers have a dual function. They form *potential fields* and thus stabilize the material structure.

A healthy organism is characterized by a high *collective coherence* of all its intelligent (!) cells. These are in a voluntary association to serve a common task. This can also be called an *integrative function*.

Illness means de-coherence, i.e. splitting off of certain areas from the functional unit and thus separation. The goal of any treatment is therefore called *re-integration*, or restoration of a high degree of coherence. Specifically, this means the reduction of chronic inflammation and normalization of cell metabolism in conjunction with the acids-base balance.

UNITED life supporting **MEDICINE ULM** is much more than just the union of naturopathy and conventional medicine. The scientific framework is not formed, as hitherto, by a natural science that acts reductionistically, linear-causally, but by quantum mechanics, which can grasp larger correlations. The previous linear findings are reinterpreted and adapted to the life processes, whereby a qualitatively higher level is achieved. Polarity replaces duality. Specialists become *generalists*. Patients are key players who are guided by the physician to gain the necessary support in their healing process.

The UNITED life supporting MEDICINE strengthens life processes by looking for and transforming the causes of disrupted regulatory processes on all levels – from psyche to soma. As long as the labile regulatory balance (homeo-dynamics) is maintained as bipolar control and thus a rapid adaptability is possible, chronic diseases are excluded. So the goal is to initiate again the inner healing process through self-regulation.

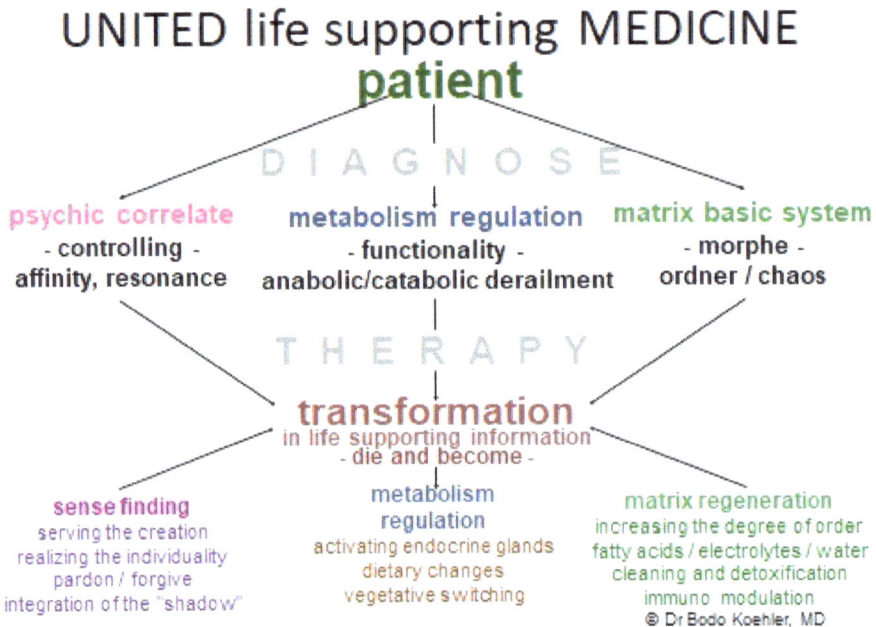

Fig.2: The UNITED life supporting MEDICINE is not only holistically oriented, but fully considers the interactions of all systems with each other. In this case, the superordinate control of matter by the spirit is given the due importance.

The provision of information is in the foreground. The structure is important for the processes and enables the function, but it constantly has to adapt to new psychic requirements. That's why the psyche ranks right up front. Emotions shape the motivation from where our actions are derived. The body follows these requirements with the regulation of cell metabolism (anabolic / catabolic), but at the same time has to respond to all external stresses that disturb its unstable equilibrium. This balancing act requires a lot of dynamism.

The scientific basics of the ULM form the following 4 main topics:
- ➢ psycho regulation, question of meaning, personal worldview
- ➢ The 3 + 1 law according to W. Pauli and the bipolar regulation
- ➢ The categorical ORDER SYSTEM – the Luescher cube
- ➢ The uniform REFERENCE SYSTEM – the cell metabolism

Psycho regulation, question of sense, personal worldview
There are a few things in life that we first have to understand, because *philosophy* (the love of wisdom) is not part of normal education, let alone upbringing. Every (!) act and thus dealing with others, but also with oneself – nutrition, lifestyle etc. – is an expression of the personal worldview. Wars would be unthinkable in a humane influence. But even illnesses would only rarely occur if a conscious, loving treatment of one's own body was cultivated.

Many diseases are based on nutritional deficiencies, lack of exercise, sleep deficits, alcohol abuse or similar. Behind all this lies the psychic self-control, which follows one (or no) sense. That is why (!) must be considerate this to every chronic disease there, both diagnostically and therapeutically. This seems to be difficult at first, because every human being is an unmistakable individual. A great help is provided by the Luescher test.

The 3 + 1 law a.t. W. Pauli and bipolar regulation
Nobel laureate Wolfgang Pauli had rediscovered the neutrino that Nicola Tesla had already described as "radiation" before him. Pauli found out by calculations that besides the 3 known elementary particles *neutron, proton* and *electron* had to belong something fourth and postulated the **neutrino**. Since it is massless and has some other properties than the other 3, but all 4 together represent the basic

building blocks of all matter, he formulated the *3 + 1 law*. This means that there are always 4 components in a system, three of which are similar and the fourth may have different properties.

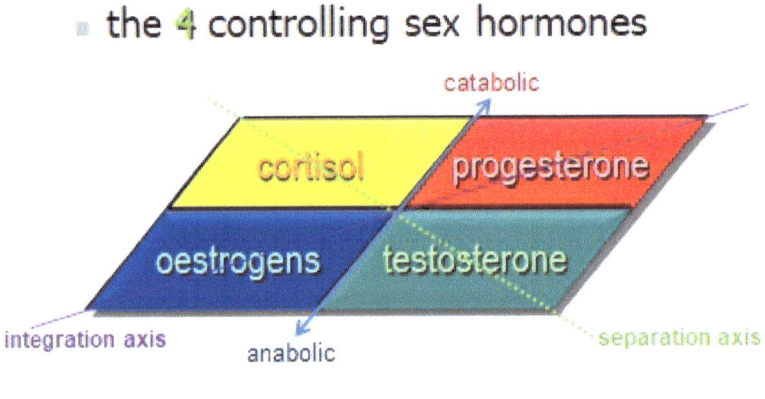

Fig.3: Using the example of the 4 sex hormones, the bipolar conditions can be displayed very well. Progesterone is the antagonist of the oestrogens and cortisol the antagonist of the testosterone. Each axle strives for a dynamic balance and thus low energy consumption.

If the functional systems are arranged in living organisms from this point of view, a surprising regularity is shown: all four components of a system are in dynamic dependence on each other, in a *crossed polarity*, with both axis are in *reciprocal relation* to each other. This means in plain language: One polarity brings out the other, or in other words: every disturbance on a polar axis is due to the other, crossed axis.

The sex hormones (Fig. 3) meet the 3 + 1 law a.t. Pauli in a classic way, as cortisol seems to make an exception. All 4 are in constant interaction. The separation axis is made possible by the axis of integration and vice versa (reciprocity). If a hormone is substituted in the case of a deficiency, this automatically affects the other three and can lead to a *counter-regulation*. This phenomenon should always be considered, because in practice, it often happens to paradoxical effects. A sedative can stimulate, rather than to sedate.

Even with the hormones, if a possible counter-regulation is not taken into account, increased blood levels of a hormone can appear even it was not substituted at all. Therefore, basically all 4 components of a system should always be determined together in order to correctly assess the 4-pole interactions.

The categorical ORDER SYSTEM has been missing in medicine so far. It is particularly important for living organisms to capture *relationships and interactions*. The 4-dimensional cube, which was initially designed by Prof Dr Max Luescher, PhD for psychology, naturally offers itself as an ordering system, because in this way the *influence of the psyche* on the 4-pole regulatory processes can be immediately read, but not only this: If a component gets into a shortcoming, then it can immediately be seen what effects it will have on the other 3 and what counter-regulation is to be expected.

For example, if there is a deficiency in a blue and / or green quadrant (anabolic weakness), catabolic counter regulation occurs in the form of tachycardia, hypertension, or the like. Anyone who sends such a patient to a cardiologist uses the wrong address. In this case, every effort must be made to strengthen the anabolic side, depending on the level at which the problem lies.

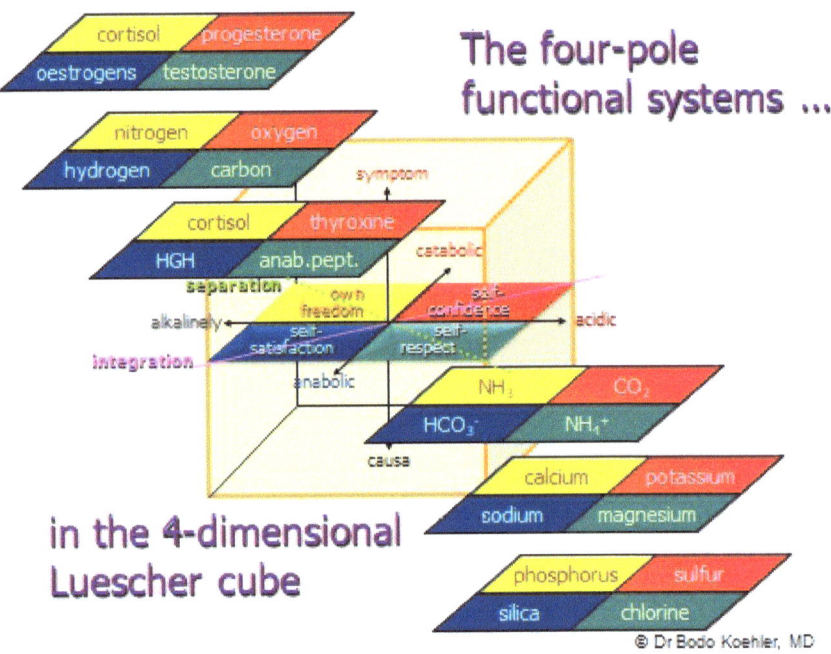

Fig.4: This selection shows the hierarchy of functional systems from the centre outwards. Changes in a quadrant, e.g. blue's *self-satisfaction* will first affect the overlying cell metabolism and underlying acids-base homeostasis and then gradually spread to the blue quadrants of all other planes.

All functional systems are hierarchically linked with each other and influence each other. The intentions of the psyche first affect cell metabolism and acids-base regulation. Later, other systems will be covered.

The uniform REFERENCE SYSTEM was also missing so far. The *cell metabolism* is virtually predestined for this because it is the focus of all branches of medicine. Each functional system is dependent on its quality, every disease manifests itself in the cell metabolism (anabolic versus catabolic derailment) and every therapy starts there.

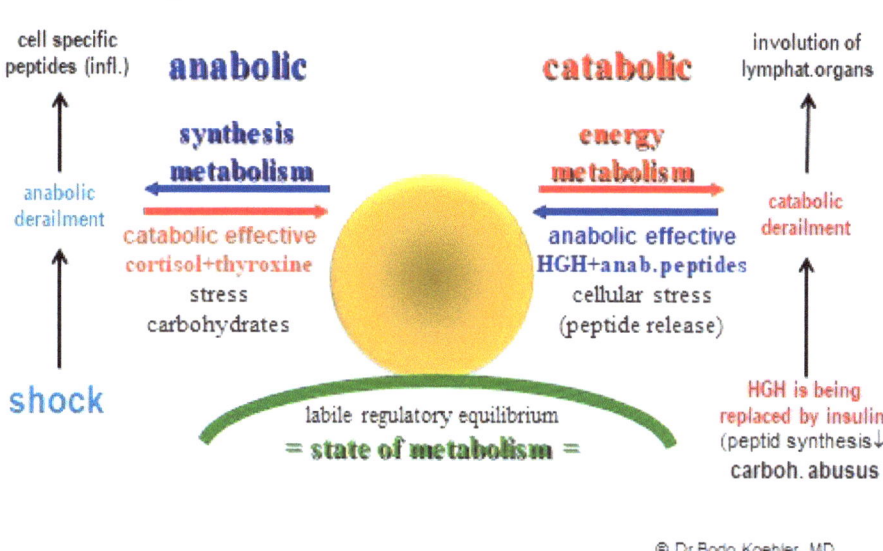

Fig.5: The bipolar regulation of cell metabolism. Anabolic peptides can replace HGH, which can be blocked by insulin as well as permanent psychic stress. However, if these remain elevated after an acute illness for a longer period of time, chronification occurs because the cortisol receptors on the nucleus are already degraded on the 8th day.

The *ability to regulate* cell metabolism (hormonal and vegetative) as a measure of health can be easily detected with bioenergetics diagnostics (for example, with MORA*nova* or ZMR 703) and is also suitable for follow-up (Fig. 11 page 32).

Responsible for the so-called "basic regulation" are electron shifts. If there are more demands, controlling hormones appear, as shown in Fig. 5.

For the understanding of the cell function and thus of every tissue the following sentence of the metabolic researcher Prof Dr Dr Juergen Schole ground-breaking:

"The cell metabolism can only regulate normally if the anabolic-acting HGH (human growth hormone) and the catabolic hormones cortisol and thyroxine are present in the cell *and* nucleus *at the same time*." (Emphasis added by the author).

Because of its central position in medicine, the *regulation of cell metabolism* is not only suitable as a diagnostic tool for emerging disorders (anabolic versus catabolic derailment), but also in an excellent way as a follow-up. The above-mentioned, non-invasive measurement methods using a multifunctional ear sensor make a quick, cost-effective assessment possible.

The resulting statements are not only important for the treatment of diseases. In particular, they are also suitable for assessing the severity, which is particularly important in cancer or other difficult to assess situations and for prevention.

As long as the cell metabolism in relation to the acids-base balance behaves dynamically, constantly regulated from one side of the polar axis to the other and back again, then the organism has the upper hand, no matter what. However, if a regulation blockage is already recognizable without any symptom; (further) diagnostic measures should be taken immediately. It's that easy!

Regulation of Cell Metabolism

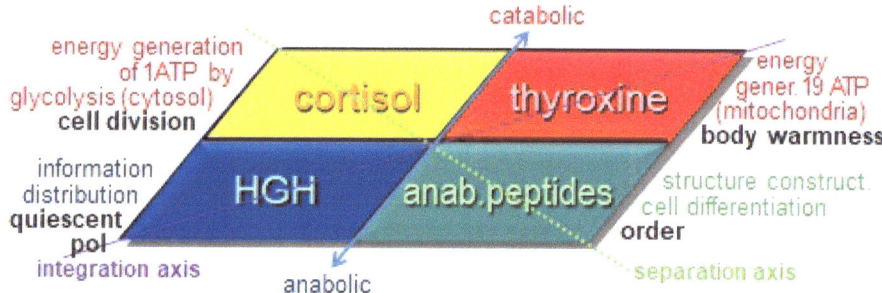

Fig.6: The regulation of cell metabolism in the usual four-pole representation. It should be noted that the (yellow-green) separation axis is controlled by the *reciprocally* arranged integration axis and vice versa.

Disturbances on one of these polar axes therefore have their cause on the other. At the edge the meaning of the quadrants for the organism is listed. In particular, the temperature-dependent mode of energy generation plays a major role. The lower limit for normal mitochondrial function is 36.5 ° C (97,7 ° F).

Pathogenesis

- **Overloading** a system (or more), e.g. through stress, or psychic shock
- **Local inflammation** (*anabolic* derailment of cell metabolism > load of focal disturbances)
- **Toxic loads** (*catabolic* derailment of the cell metabolism > permanent stress)
- **Deficiency states** versus overloading (nutrition)

These are the 4 main points that must always be remembered, because they are the ones that can disturb the *labile regulatory balance* and prevent a balance. The resulting permanent imbalance leads to one-sided loads that cannot be sustained in the long term. Either the *father principle* is disturbed or the *mother principle* (see under Therapy).

Excessive demand
The resilience of a functional system depends on the constitution and thus on genetics and epigenetics. These should be considered as a priority. However, any overload depends above all on the intent behind it, i.e. it is self-made and an expression of the individual state of consciousness. The diabetic will only develop symptoms if he has a constantly high consumption of easily usable carbohydrates – only then! The diabetic could, however, have normal sugar levels despite being fed the wrong amount of carbohydrates if he would be charged accordingly.

Underload has the same disease severity as overtaxing, no matter which organ system it refers to. Above all, there is a lack of exercise. Even dementia could be improved by dosed physical training.

The *psychic shock* is a special feature in this context. It leads to an immediate anabolic derailment of one or more functional systems, which can lead to a chronic inflammation.

Chronic inflammation
Any acute defence reaction can become chronic. The healing process is controlled by the brain (hormonal and via vegetative nervous system). It is genetically determined, for a 7-day acute phase (alarm reaction according to Hans Selye) and then 3 weeks convalescence.

The cortisol receptors on the cell nucleus are degraded again on the 8th day. If, however, the anabolic peptides predominate in the cell, chronic inflammation occurs, as catabolic counter regulation is no longer possible.

The reason for the suspension is an existing lack of regulators (HGH, thyroxine, cortisol), because then the acute phase cannot be intense enough (for example with a high fever). Possible insufficiencies should first be clarified by examining the associated endocrine glands (adrenals, thyroid and pituitary gland).

Toxic loads
Detoxification (including sweating) is a catabolic process. Excessive poisoning, especially over long periods of time, overstrains the catabolic part of the cell metabolism and the excretory organs, in particular the liver and kidneys. Here it is not enough to strengthen only the function of the mitochondria, but it is intensive relief measures required, especially on the intestines and liver / bile, while restraining with food intake, up to fasting.
In order to get rid of the toxic loads in a direct way, the matrix regeneration therapy with the MRT 503 is particularly suitable.

Mineral powder from *volcanic rock* has also proven its worth, because it prevents the re-uptake of poisons that are excreted in the intestine with bile. *Curcuma*, which as bittern besides many other positive effects also stimulates the bile function, has a supporting effect here. A tried and tested remedy for many years is CurSiMag®, which also contains *magnesium citrate* in addition to the substances mentioned.

Deficiency states versus overloading
Nutrition issues primarily affect the liver metabolism. Each one-sidedness leads to deficiencies; each over load also creates problems. The non-alcoholic fatty liver (even in the case of slimness) attacks (in addition to the alcoholic liver disease) more and more and is the trigger of many serious sequelae, among others cardiovascular, diabetes, but also cancer. Short fasting sessions can be very helpful. Even 1 fasting day a week (for example, fermented vegetable juice fasting) is used to relieve the liver.

However, the main reason for fat deposition in the various organs is not in the fat intake, but in too many readily available carbohydrates that are converted into fat (triglycerides) in the liver with insulin participation.

Another aspect arises from the blood groups that are genetically predetermined. Depending on their affiliation, there may be a beneficial or debilitating influence on the immune system. For example, BG A representatives are born vegetarians, whereas BG 0 are meat eaters. Further information can be found in the specified literature.

Psycho regulation
All 4 points are dominated by the *mental mood*. Therefore, the focus should be on diagnosis and therapy.

Without knowing the deeper reason behind every action and ultimately overburdening / underburdening, cannot be treated causally.

To diagnose a person correctly is not an easy task. The Chinese have already dealt with this problem 5,000 years ago. The 5 phases of conversion (formerly called 5 elements) bring a structure into the interactions of psyche and soma.

Max Luescher attributed the different behaviours to four self-esteems: *personal contentedness, self-respect, self-confidence, personal freedom.*

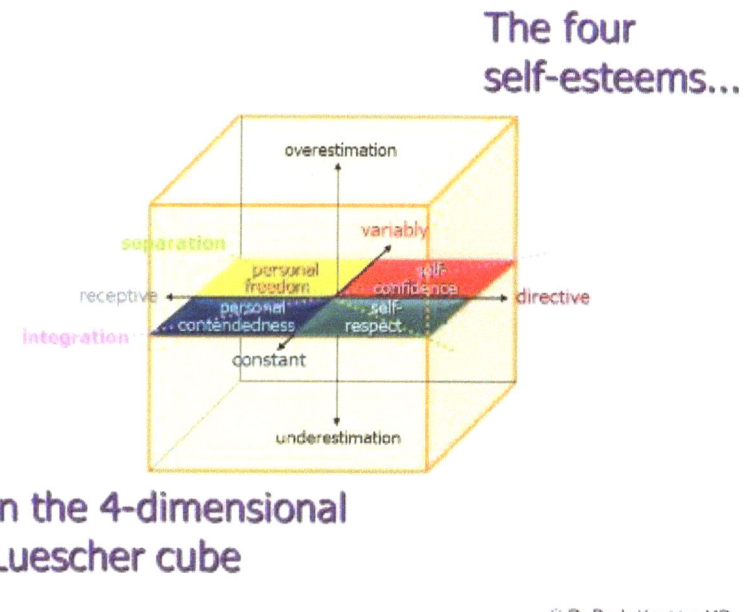

Fig.7: The Luescher cube and the 4 self-esteems. Only when all 4 are realized can we live in *harmony*. Harmony is the balance of all polar opposites.

The connection of psycho regulation with the various functional systems has already been shown in Fig. 4. It cannot be emphasized enough that the reason for any loss of function of one or more systems is always and without exception (!) in psycho regulation, which reflects the state of consciousness. Insufficiently developed self-esteems lead to an overvaluation or underestimation of reality with incorrect perception and resulting mistakes.

Reciprocity
The visible is produced by the invisible. In the background of visible reality, countless energetic interactions occur. They are the actual effectors and control our world of experience. Against this background, the following explanations can be better understood.

Everything is related to everything, as we have learned from quantum physics. But it is subject to a high hierarchical order, which is why not every influence can be effective. To this order belongs the law of reciprocity, which can be represented in the Luescher cube.

Mathematically speaking, reciprocity means that about emotions an information that is infinitely spread in the background field (potential field, spirit) is retrieved and, by inversion, focuses on one point. This can be represented geometrically as a line onto which another line is projected as a point, creating a cross. The formula is $1/x$, so it's a proportion, a ratio.

This old school knowledge (!) has a great significance for us. In fact, we can understand much better what the real cause behind the individual symptoms is and start specific treatment there.

As can be seen in Fig. 7, the two polar axes of integration and separation stand perpendicular to each other. They are thus in a reciprocal relationship to each other, which means that the polarity of one axis is reflected at the other (punctiform) and thus influences this.
More dramatically, it can be formulated that a disturbance of the axis of integration (as a symptom) shows on the separation axis and vice versa. Or formulated positively: One axis can only regulate normally, when the other axis is balanced.

This requires a "collective coherence". By this is meant that all cells and tissues have joined together to serve a common purpose. An intelligent act!

Many misunderstandings and misdiagnosis of diseases are based on a mechanistic view of the body. Only through quantum mechanics *consciousness* came into play, because life is to be understood only as an intelligent consequence of rhythmic processes.

Coherence is based on two opposing processes: the pursuit of the "quantum mechanical ground state" as a calming pole on the one hand and high dynamics on the other. In the ground state (according to Dr Bernd Zeiger, PhD), the *inverted* 3rd law of thermodynamics has an effect, which automatically increases the *internal order* of a system.

This "haven of peace" (quiescent pole) can be proven on different levels, depending on which system is considered. For the cell it is the nucleus and for the whole organism it is the kidneys. They form a functional unit (integration axis) with the heart.

Disease can therefore be equated with loss of coherence. The associated increased energy consumption reduces resources, which leads to fatigue in the long term.

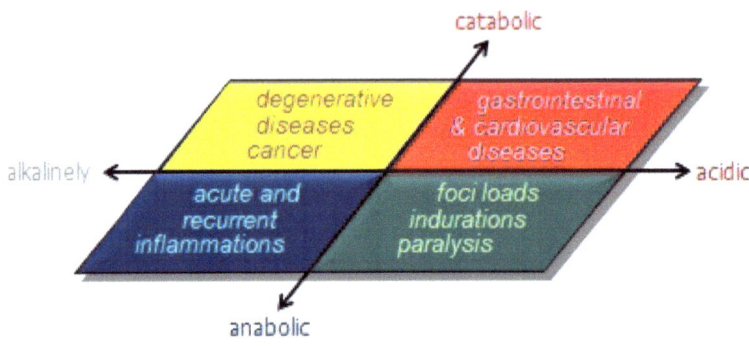

Fig.8: All diseases can be assigned to the 4 quadrants. This not only makes it easier to identify the cause, but also to derive a deeply effective therapy from it.

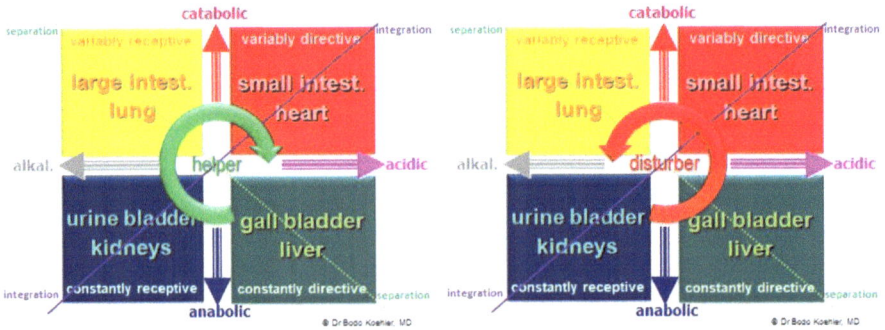

Fig.9 a + b: Interactions of organ systems

What has not yet been clarified is the question of which pole of the respective polar axes is the problem (usually as a lack). There is another principle of order, namely the law of conversion, as the old Chinese have already stated. This is what the organ clock is derived from. Clockwise is the normal circulation; in the counter clockwise direction disturbances can occur.

In conjunction with Figures 8 and 9, this means:
- ➢ Recurrent inflammations (blue) are caused by yellow (functional circuit large intestine / lung). Blue is however supported by green (functional circuit bile/liver). Green stands for high order, firmness and authenticity as well as *self-respect* (> self-love!)
- ➢ Disturbance fields, induration, paralyzes, e.g. MS (green) have their cause in the blue (bladder / kidney functional circuit). Green is however supported by red (functional circuit small intestine / heart). Red stands for dynamism, resolution, movement, but above all *self-confidence.*
- ➢ Gastrointestinal and cardiovascular diseases, infarction, apoplexy (red) have their cause in the green (functional circuit bile / liver). Red is however supported by yellow (functional circuit large intestine / lung). Yellow stands for openness, new beginnings, letting go and *personal freedom.*
- ➢ Degenerative diseases up to cancer (yellow) have their cause in the red (functional circuit small intestine / heart). Yellow is supported by blue (bladder / kidneys). Blue stands for primal trust, relationships, commitment, but also *personal contentedness.*

That makes a lot of sense and opens up completely new perspectives on the pathogenesis. Under "Therapy" the resulting possibilities are presented.

Diagnostics

- **Anamnesis** (see questionnaire below)

- **Personality diagnostics** (Luescher-Test / Psycho Kinesiology PK / PSE)
- **Bioenergetics testing** with MORA*nova* / Decoder, VEGA-DFM or -Expert, EAV / Resonance Test / Kinesiology, HRV
- **Imaging procedures** (sonography, X-ray, CT, MRI)

- **laboratory tests**

Case history

The collection of data by an anamnesis is underestimated in importance. It is usually the first doctor-patient encounter, during which a deep bond of trust should build up. Typing the information into the computer, without eye contact, is not only completely counterproductive, but also gives the chance of an emotional encounter in which the crucial healing information can be exchanged (Fig. 10). The holistic doctor also reads between the lines and follows his intuition. Then he often knows even before evaluating the examination findings what a patient actually lacks and is only confirmed by the results.

Of course, this does not succeed under time pressure. The talking medicine is therefore given more space in the UNITED MEDICINE. But this is primarily about a non-verbal communication, which takes place in silence, so in the pauses. The necessary rest and intensive eye contact are simultaneously anxiolytic. In the patients who had such an encounter with the doctor, the healing process begins on the way home, because the necessary information for the renewed initiation of stagnant life processes was retrieved from the spirit and can take effect immediately. Quite often it happens that patients when leaving the practice say: "Doctor, thank you, I'm already much better!"

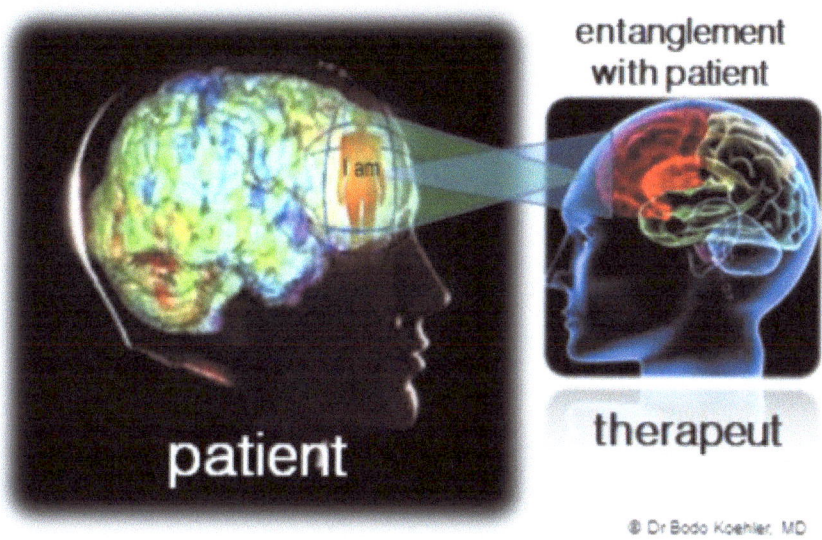

Fig.10: Generation of the healing information in the frontal brain of the patients by mirror neurons.

Questionnaire for the case history
- ☐ permanent psychic stress? Tendency to depression?
- ☐ partner problems, children, relationship?
- ☐ accidents, injuries, concussion?
- ☐ poison exposure, narcosis?
- ☐ hair dye? Deo?
- ☐ amalgam fillings?
- ☐ high consumption of mercury-contaminated fish?
- ☐ dealing with electro-smog?
- ☐ mould exposure?
- ☐ continuous intake of harmful drugs?

- ☐ proton pump inhibitors? Statins?
- ☐ smoking?
- ☐ sleeping habits?
- ☐ fulfilling sexuality?
- ☐ snoring?
- ☐ oral hygiene?
- ☐ implants of any kind?
- ☐ existing chronic diseases?
- ☐ Lime disease?
- ☐ chronic sinusitis?
- ☐ frequent angina?
- ☐ strain with EBV, chlamydia, herpes?
- ☐ food habits: mixed food? Diets? Vegan?
- ☐ drinking habits? Alcohol?
- ☐ blood type?
- ☐ predominantly organic food or industrial food?
- ☐ heated oils (trans fats) in the food?
- ☐ many carbohydrates?
- ☐ indigestion? Fat intolerance?
- ☐ stool habits? Colour?
- ☐ sweating – more often or rarely?
- ☐ exercise habits? Lot of sitting? Sports?

Personality Assessment

Taking into account the various access routes to the genetic determined constitution of health and psycho regulation, it is possible to work out a picture that is not only important for the doctor, but also provides access to the underlying problems of the patients. The individual methods are discussed in more detail in the big *textbook*.

The following points are groundbreaking:

- Luescher test
- Determination of HDL cholesterol (> 70 pathological)
- Relation Oxytocin – ADH
- thyroid diagnosis
- Determination of the 4 neuromodulators (Saliva)
- Stool diagnostics!
- Antibody determination of neuro-viruses (herpes etc.)
- Relation D-hormone active / inactive (receptors!)

Bioenergetics testing

It is in all test procedures to capture the disease with its interactions. The basic scheme is provided by the 4 disease groups, as shown in Fig. 8 p. 26. A specific hierarchy must be observed: All (!) diseases begin in the blue quadrant (acute inflammation with defence reaction). This can lead to a chronification on the anabolic side (green quadrant, disturbance field disease), or to a switch to the catabolic side. Then it comes either to degeneration up to malignant developments, or sudden events such as stroke, heart attack, etc. Also the massive running gastrointestinal diseases such as ulcers, diverticulitis or ileus belong there. Leading the way is the condition of the milieu (acidic or alkaline).

On this scientific background, which we owe to the metabolic research of J. Schole, the ZMR device 703 is based and, more recently, the 4-pole diagnose module in the MORA*nova*. Both offer the advantage of fully automatic measurement with subsequent therapy based on it.

Indirect indications, especially load by disturbance fields, are provided by Decoder, VEGA-Expert, thermography and other bioenergetics devices f.e., HRV, but also kinesiological tests or the Biotensor. It is not only important to recognize what is, but what does not regulate.

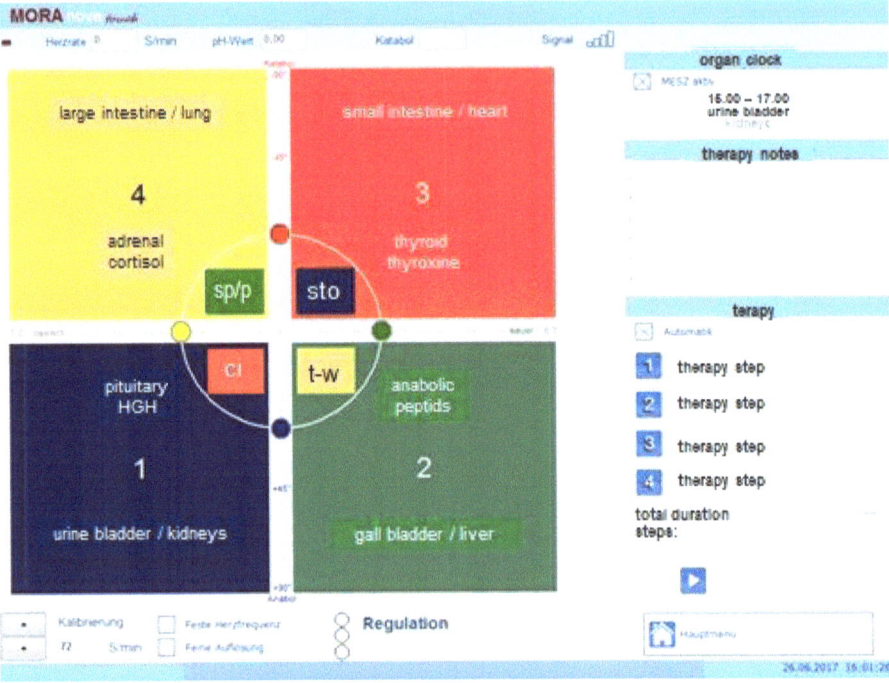

Fig.11: Monitor image of the 4-pole regulation of cell metabolism in conjunction with the acids-base balance. The 4 Luescher colours refer to the higher positioned psycho regulation. You can see the ground state, where all 4 colour points are on the inner circle. For the assessment, however, it is not a normal "state" that is crucial, but the dynamics in the adaptation to changing environmental influences, which is reflected in the movement around the middle position.

Imaging procedures

The statements we get from ultrasonography, x-rays, etc. are usually overestimated. A NAFLD (fatty liver disease) usually does *not* (yet) show up in ultrasound. Arthritis with severe pain does *not* have to be seen in X-ray. Many people walk around with degenerated hip joints,

but *without* pain. It is *impossible* to tell about a tumour whether it has been standing still (perhaps for years) or is growing aggressively.
Very often the symptoms differ from the local findings! Therefore the sentence applies:

From the shape cannot be concluded on the function!

Laboratory analyses

- **cell metabolism** (3 endocrine glands {cortisol stress profile, IGF-1 and 3, thyroid gland*) sex hormones
- **4 neuro transmitters** {dopamine, epinephrine, acetylcholine, serotonin}
- **fasting blood sugar**; **Insulin, HbA1c, homocysteine**
- **large blood count**, erythrocyte sedimentation (ionization energy!), electrophoresis
- **liver function**, **renal function**,
- **inflammation** (hs-CRP, IL-6, TNF-α)
- **vitamins** (B group, D-hormone active / inactive)
- **minerals** (Pot., Mag., Sod., Ca, Cu, Zn, Se, Iodine)
- **total cholesterol**, HDL, LDL,
- **Estronex test** (to determine the liver detoxification pathways)
- **large stool diagnostics** (special laboratories reserved)

Special features and standard values
From the obtained values cannot be concluded on the function! This can only be done by functional tests, e.g. exercise ECG. This also applies to the thyroid, which would require a daily profile.

*) Thyroid: T_3 3.2-4.4 ng / l; free T_4 (storage form) 9.3-17 ng / l
Ratio T_4 / T_3 4 : 1; TSH (+/- 1.0)
reverse T_3 (< 200 pg / ml) inhibits free T_3,
Ratio free T_3 x 100 / reverse T_3: > 2

estradiol 50-250 ng / l; progesterone 1-20 mg / ml
Ratio of estradiol / progesterone: 1:10

total testosterone 500-1000 mg / dl; free testosterone 6.5-18 mg / dl
    cortisol in the morning 10-18 mcg / dl
    pregnenolol 50-100 µg / l
    DHEA-S 3.5-4.3 mg / l woman
        4.0-5.0 mg / l man

    Cu minus 3x coeruloplasmin < 30
    Zn 900-1200 µg / l (serum), in whole blood 600-750 µg / dl;
    Ratio Cu / Zn: 0.8-1.0

    Mg 1.2-1.7 mmol / l in whole blood
    Se 110-150 µg / l

Ratio of omega-6 / omega-3 in the blood: 0.5-3
(not < 0.5 >>> bleeding)

Ratio of albumin (> 55 g / l) / globulin in the blood: > 1.8

Inflammatory markers: hs-CRP < 0.9 mg / l
        IL-6 < 3 ng / l
        TNF-α < 8.0 pg / ml
        C4A < 2830 ng / ml
        TGF-β1 < 2380 pg / ml
        MSH (melanocyte-stim. horm.) 35-81 pg/ml
        Urine test for mycotoxins

glutathione (GSH) 5.0-5.5 µmol / l

glucose (fasting)   60 - 90 mg / dl
Insulin   2.5 - 25 mU / l
HbA1c   4   - 6%; 20-40 mmol / molHb

    vit. E   12-20 mcg / ml
    vit. B1   50-75 µg / l (whole blood); 20-30 µmol/l (serum)
    vit. B6   20-30 µg / l (whole blood)
    vit. B9 (folate) 15-25 ng / ml (whole blood)
    vit. B12   500-770 pg / ml (whole blood)

    vit. D3   20-50 µg / l (25-OH-D3 pre-hormone)
                    50-120 nmol / l
    D-hormone   15-20 pg / ml (1,25-dihydroxy-D2)
                    30-50 nmol / l

Cyrex Array 20 = negative (measure of open blood-brain barrier)
Cyrex Array 3 = negative (gluten intolerances)
Cyrex Array 4 = negative (allergy: rye, barley, sesame, oats, rice)
Cyrex Array 5 = negative (numerous auto-antibodies)

Auto-antibodies are formed against AGEs. AGEs produce free radicals, activate inflammation, and open the blood - brain barrier

IDE (insulin-degrading enzyme insulysin)
also breaks down beta-amyloid!

Neuropsychological test: MoCA (www.mocatest.org),
Norm 26-30; < 19 = dementia

Example of a laboratory order
IGF-1 and 3
TSH
reverse and free T_3
free T_4

estradiol
pregnenolol
estrol
progestogene
free testosterone
DHEAS

homocysteine
hs-CRP
fasten blood sugar + Insulin
HbA1c
electrophoresis
IL-6
TNF-α

B vitamins 1, 6, 9, 12
"vitamin" D active (hormone) and inactive (precursor),
minerals in whole blood: Pot., Mag, Cu, Zn

serum minerals: Sod., Ca, Se, Zn, Cu

erythrocite sedimentation
large blood count,
GOT
GPT
Gamma-GT
AP
total cholesterol, HDL
creatinine
GFR

cortisol stress profile
neuromodulators (dopamine, epinephrine, acetylcholine, serotonin)
Estronex test

Therapy

First and foremost, it is important to enable the organism to produce its own dynamic equilibrium in all functional systems again. These are controlled bipolar, that means over a crossed polarity. This enables a high dynamic without jeopardizing the overall order of the system. One of these polarities is named after the assignment in the Luescher cube as *integration axis*, the other as a *separation axis*. Here is the law of reciprocity. By this is meant that the normal function of one axis is ensured by the other, perpendicular axis (Fig.7 page 23).

If the polarities are overloaded on one side, this can create a duality. This means that "as-well-as" changes into "either-or", what exclusion means. This automatically leads to too much on the one hand and too little on the other hand. Overcrowding on the one hand and lack on the other are inevitable. A chronic disease indicates that the organism can not return to an ordered dynamic by itself.

As already explained in the chapter "Reciprocity" on page 24, the 4 quadrants influence each other mutually, following a fixed order. Clockwise is *assisted*, counter clockwise may cause *disturbances* (Figure 9 p. 26). It is usually so that not the surplus – the excess – is the cause (but can produce the symptoms!), but the lack. For this reason, the treatment consistently follows this pattern and corrects the derailed polarity in the background by the weaker pole is balanced with the stronger.

All features of the various levels of a pole are used, from the colour itself to the psychic equivalent, the self-esteem of M. Luescher.

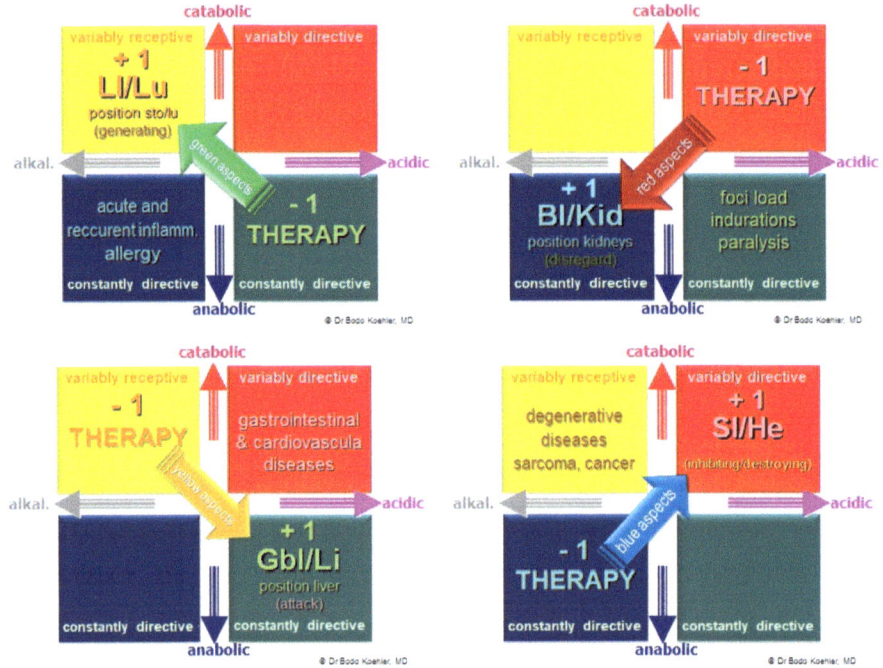

Fig.12: The therapy principle of the 4 quadrants according to the rules of TCM (5 conversion phases). With bioelectronics devices such as the ZMR 703 and the diagnostic module of the MORA*nova*, a treatment can be fully automatic.

The arrows always point to the disturbing quadrant and indicate that the "healthy" pole on the same axis is used to compensate for the shortage.

Mother and father principle

In conformity to the life processes should be therapeutically attempted to "mother" a disturbed father principle and vice versa a disturbed mother principle to "fatherize".

Under "mother principle" all feminine aspects are subsumed, i.e. *openness, calm, primal trust, overview, receiving, caring, intuition* – and also right brain, the sensor system as well as the hormone system.

Accordingly, all male aspects are attributed to the "father principle" and thus *concentration, logical thinking* (left hemisphere), *stimulation, enforcement* (directive) and the controlling nervous system.

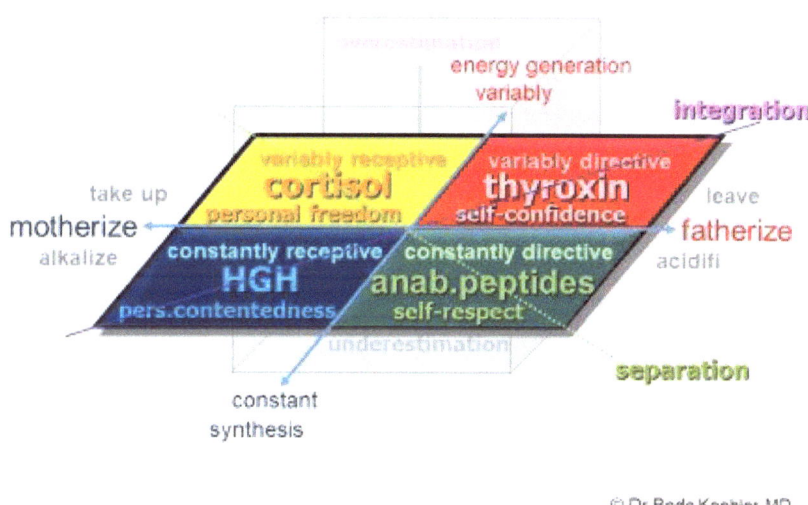

Fig.13: The principle of polar equalization can be understood very well in this illustration. No matter on which level – integration and separation axes always have to be balanced.

Both principles are suitable for balancing of the four-pole regulation. So if the directive male principle is too weak (in red or green) it has to be fatherized, when the receptive female principle is too weak (in blue or yellow), must be mothered.

In concrete terms, this means (compare Fig.8, p. 26 and Fig.13 p. 39):
- ➢ Acute and recurrent inflammation must be *fatherized*
- ➢ Indurations and paralysis must be *mothered*
- ➢ Cardiovascular and gastrointestinal diseases *as well*
- ➢ Degeneration and malignant diseases must in turn be *fatherized.*

Since every change always starts from the spiritual, the consciousness work of the patients is at the forefront. This means that **inflammation / allergy** (blue) often follows on suppressed emotional needs (- - 2). That is why the active shaping of life is important. Above all, that means **self-love**. Finally do the things that are good for your own SELF!

In patients with **disturbance fields** or even paralysis (green) is often a denial of learning processes (- - 3) in the foreground. They should develop **activity** and make peace with the past to get out of their contraction. The motto is: Up to new deeds!

Cardiovascular or gastrointestinal disorders (red) lack the rhythm with the necessary rest periods. They often suffer from loss of reality, which can result in futility (- - 4). This is about an **expansion of consciousness**, so that the lost contact with the spiritual origin can be restored.

Patients with **degeneration up to cancer disease** (yellow) should develop a sense of community (coherence) and become aware of the connection of everything to everything. It is often about loss of trust and relationship (- -1) and lost **primal trust**. It is important to find the quiescent pole in the quantum mechanical ground state and to live it out.

The cohesion in the body is generated via the integration axis blue-red. The task for all regulatory processes is to maintain *collective coherence*, or to restore it after any exposure to toxins, microbes or mental stress. Prerequisite is a stable quiescent pole (the kidneys) as the basis for a high metabolic dynamics, which depends on the thyroid gland.

Since all healing processes are controlled by the brain and monitored via the nervous system, a treatment focused on that is paramount. It should not be forgotten, however, that these are predominantly unconscious processes and only "land" 4% in day consciousness. For this reason, the empathic encounter (see Fig. 10 page 29) is so crucial in which the unconscious healing information crystallizes out in the brain of the patient via mirror neurons. That cannot do any other good therapy.
The unconscious is also reached with the Luescher test, which is why it is so valuable for personality diagnostics.

Coherence therapy CHT is the logical consequence of the previously known scientific basics. Since collective coherence needs a quiescent pole to be able to return to the quantum mechanical ground state again and again after every stress, the kidneys are of particular importance. These correspond with the heart on the axis of integration. Together, they are responsible for the re-integration of separated areas (e.g. foci of inflammation).

The preparation proceeds as follows (Fig. 14): The interference field information is routed via the neck electrode of the headphones (NEC 708) to the Limbic system. This activates the feeling underlying the illness via resonance. The frontal brain, will be informed about the theta waves generated by the brain, and adequately answers the emotions (will, intention). This impulse is lead to the kidneys, the location of the life information. These are in constant interaction with the heart via the axis of integration. The heart gets transmitted the disturbance field information with the hand applicator of the MRT 503, after having passed through the "harmony cell" in the device. As a result, chaotic disturbance field information meets *already transformed* interference field information. The transcendental aspect of the heart is thereby able to transform the separative disturbance information into integrative (love), which restores the healthy state of collective coherence.

The interfering field itself is used (only) as a reference for the therapeutic success. If there are several interference fields, these can be activated during the treatment and react.

The treatment can be done once a week without additional therapy steps. In acute cases (such as severe pain) more often.

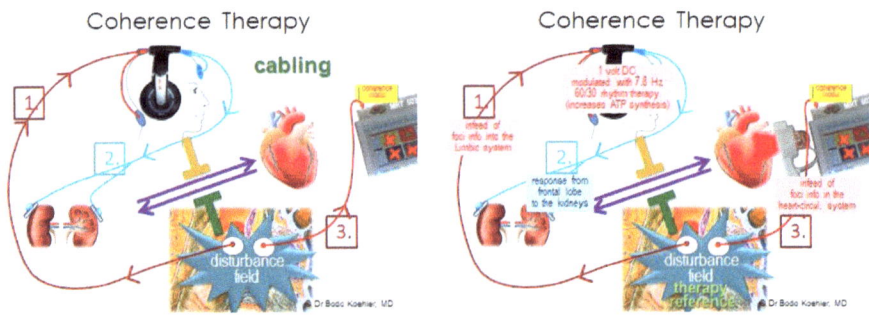

Fig.14: Since reality is fundamentally switched via emotions, the transformation of stressful situations and emotions stored (!) in the interference field is a *conditio sine qua non* for the healing process. In addition to the MRT 503 and the NEC 708 headphones, a special cable set is required to perform the treatment.

Whoever has understood the principle can perform the treatment as meditation, since is treated here according to the higher *spiritual law of love*.

Balancing therapy with Equalizer EQ 103
This new therapy instrument EQ 103 simplifies the treatment considerably, since it is small and transportable. It includes some extra properties, e.g. wireless transmission of information with pure light, but without (!) electro-smog, and also analogous storage of the body signal. Indispensable, however, are the 4 regulators of cell metabolism, which are also integrated.

Because this form of therapy opens up completely new possibilities, it is described in more detail here.
The *Equalizer EQ 103* can be used to *compensate* for existing information gaps in the light processing of our body, caused by chronic stress – material or psychological.

The device has the following *features:*
- white full spectrum light for information acquisition
- red light (λ 630nm) stimulates the cell, nucleus & mitochondria
- infrared light for deep regeneration
- white noise (all frequencies are included)
- dynamic magnetic field, modulated with biological signals
- scalar field, especially for coupling to the quantum field
- 7.83 Hz modulation (Schumann; resonance with hippocampus)
- DC application (compensation of charge differences)
- Subtraction Neutralization Therapy SNT
- Optional inversion of the input signal (detoxification)
- integrated cup (can be equipped with healing information)
- Input for external signals (e.g. sounds, music, information from ZMR / Vortex, MRT)

Photons (light) are the *information carrier No. 1*. All control processes in the organism are generated via real and virtual photons. Deficiency or loss of these meaningful light particles can lead to functional failures or even serious chronic diseases. *Lack of light also means lack of sun,* because food alone is not enough for the body's needs. This requires the entire spectrum of the sun, from UV to infrared.

The *Equalizer EQ 103* has a wide range of applications, because without exception there are light and therefore information *deficits* in every illness. It is always about a deficiency caused by an imbalance that needs to be remedied.

The application can be done while sitting or lying down and is divided into 6-9 stages, which are all used one after the other, or only a selection, depending on the disease.

Therapy variants with Equalizer 103
- Cleaning the receiving channel (trauma treatment)
- Balancing the bladder meridian
- Balancing the Chakra system
- Sympathetic-parasympathetic balancing
- Balancing of side differences (pain treatment)
- Focus projection (pain treatment)
- Partner therapy
- Shock resolution
- Toxin removal, resolution of receptor blockages

Additional information can be run during the treatment, which is placed in the integrated entrance cup (coherence module, metabolic information, etc.).

Based on the fact that all *life information is of a spiritual nature* and the subtle soul is effective as a *medium* so that it can be transferred to the gross body, special emphasis is placed on *providing information*.

For this purpose, the skin area above a symptom or directly at the focus of the disease is stimulated by white, multi-frequency light, which increases the radiation of information-carrying photons. The white light is modulated with the retroreflective photons of the tissue, thereby recording the information about the locally disrupted order (duration 3 seconds). The spin of these photons – and thus the information – is stored in the device in an *analogue* manner.

The stored information is used to modulate *red* light with a wavelength of 630 nm and to irradiate it in certain skin zones. These react to the stress information of the diseased area with a defence reaction (stimulus reaction) by transforming disharmonious (polarity not balanced) oscillations into harmonic ones. This calms the system as a prerequisite for self-healing (quantum mechanical ground state QMG).

The following **key points** may be helpful for the **LSM therapy**:
- Empathic encounter, shock solution, PK, NLP
- metabolic correction, CHT, MRT 503, MORA*nova*, EQ 103
- nature-identical hormone balancing
- ketogenic diet
- orthomol. therapy (B 6 {pyridoxal-5-phosphate} 60-100nmol/l
    B 9 {methylfolate} 10-**25**ng / ml)
    B12 {**methyl**cobalamin} 600-1500pg / ml
    K 2 (Glucosa-K2®)
    CurSiMag® 2x / day
    Resveratrol 100mg / die
    Neptune™ krill oil
    Zn (e.g., in meat, oysters)

The suggestions are only stimulations. The selection depends on the blood findings or bioenergetics testing.

Lifestyle
- meaning of life, life task
- diet (more often ketogenic diet, 1 fasting day / week)
- exercise / strength training (up to 40 min./day)
- sleep (7-9 hours / 18° C = 64,4° F room temp. / full darkened)

Sense of life, life task
Anyone who walks through life without orientation not only misses the best opportunities, but does not live properly. We should see ourselves as spiritual beings, with a great potential of possibilities that we can creatively implement. It is in the nature of man that happiness and satisfaction can only be achieved through self-produced results.

For a sick person who has not set himself a task and does not see any sense in his life, the (intelligent!) cells of his immune system have absolutely no reason to work hard to successfully complete a healing process! For this reason, the personal world view of doctor and patient has a lot to do with a successful therapy.

Enough space should be found the entire creation in the personal view. If we want to achieve something, then the result is to be understood in return from our environment. Any money earned is such a return. Only if we make enough efforts, success and satisfaction can be expected. Money calms, but does not make happy. Happiness results from service, unconditional giving and love. Therefore, even the penniless can be happy, often more than the rich.

Unfortunately, the underlying law of *giving and giving back* is far too disregarded, or it is not known at all. But we can assume that there is no (!) patient who has strictly followed it. Since it is always about the balance of incriminating disharmony, and at all levels, this topic is imperative for each therapy and in the patient talk.

Nutrition
The basic knowledge of nutrition should be conscientiously studied in the "The Textbook for the UNITED life supporting MEDICINE" or the "Guide for joy of life in the best of health". The findings presented here are based on the cell metabolism – the *general reference system*, and are therefore scientifically sound and not statistical results, as used in the DGE (German Society for Nutrition).

The following table was similar published in the book "The Alzheimer Revolution" by Dr Dale E. Bredesen, MD. This should not be surprising because, first, it agrees with the findings of J. Schole and secondly, an intact nervous system is indispensable for any healing process. So what has worked well for Alzheimer's or other types of dementia is good for any brain. It has also been shown that in all degenerative diseases (up to cancer!) excessive consumption of carbohydrates is in front.

Dale Bredesen had contact with Dr Steven R. Gundry, MD, who has published the book "Bad Vegetables". Even parts of his remarks have flowed in, but were not adopted uncritically.

Regrettably, only a few experts know about the principles of cell metabolism. Therefore, there are always errors in the interpretation of effects of certain substances on the human body.

Unfortunately, it is also overlooked that all regulatory processes are bipolar and these four-pole systems are networked with each other. Here and in the textbook is therefore increasingly pointed out.

Rough division of food & beverages

often (Bio only)	less common	never
resistant starch, e.g. swedes, Egyptian rice bran, millet mushrooms	high-starch vegetables, e.g. potatoes, pumpkin, Basmati rice, semisweet fruit coconut blossom sugar, honey	sugar and all simple carbohydrates including bread, pasta, cakes, biscuits sweets, lemonade artificial sweeteners!
cauliflower, Brussels sprouts red cabbage & cabbage, kale, avocado green leafy vegetables, e.g. spinach, salads	peas, beans, broccoli, Amaranth, Quinoa, Chia solanaceae: eggplant, paprika, tomato	kohlrabi (due to phosphate) conventional cereals of all kinds, including corn unfermented soy
lemons, limes green apples, rhubarb, plantains cacao, cinnamon,	grapefruit non-tropical fruits with low glycemic index, e.g. berries, grapes, plums	sweet fruit, e.g. melon, mango, papaya
Bittern (Amara), e.g. artichokes, radicchio rocket, chicory		
asparagus, celery, fennel		
Wild fish, especially salmon, mackerel, anchovies, herring, sardines	fish from aquaculture	highly mercury-loaded fish, e.g. tuna, shark, swordfish
eggs from organic farming	organic beef, game	from factory farming
butter, cream sweet & sour buttermilk, whey, yogurt	goat's milk, sheep's milk and their products	cow's milk, milk powder conventional dairy products
ginger, chili, turmeric, black pepper, rosemary		
herbs: mint, parsley, cloves, caraway, thyme		
Prebiotics, e.g. leek		finished products, chips
sulphurous vegetables, e.g. onions, garlic		
Beverages: herbal tea, black tea, green tea low mineral water	coffee beer, wine (in moderation) winter red, summer white	hard drinks
iodinated algae, e.g. Kelp	Iodized salt, sea salt	chemical blackboard salt
walnuts, Brazil nuts, almonds	hazelnuts	peanuts! cashew
olive oil, linseed oil, perilla oil, chia oil		rapeseed oil, safflower oil, sunflower oil
ghee coconut oil	palm fat	heated oils, deep-fried, trans fats (emulsifiers)

Note the effects of combinations. For example, the simultaneous intake of fat reduces the absorption of sugar into the blood. Cream cake is therefore less problematic than a fruit cake.
In general, saturated fats are apt to increase satiety quickly, which automatically limits food intake. They may also be heated without any problems, which is not the case with oils, because it can form the Alzheimer's toxin 4-Hydroxy-Nenonal (HNE).

Attention should be paid to lectins, the so-called sticky proteins in cereals and vegetables. These pest repellents can also harm people in excess. This includes the well-known gluten as well as thousands of others. This affects especially nightshade plants such as zucchini, tomatoes, peppers, which incidentally also contain Solamine (a neurotoxin). By cooking in a pressure cooker, however, these substances are harmless.
Lectins bind to sugar and are thus passed through the intestinal wall. That's another reason why a sugar waiver is worthwhile.

A bigger problem can be caused by WGA, an agglutinin in the shell of wheat grain. It is similar to insulin and can cause autoimmune diseases, but also lead to receptor block and thus to brain shrinkage! Wheat should therefore be avoided at all costs, or used only (rarely) as extract flour.

Attention: Through gene manipulation lectins are deliberately introduced into the vegetables!

But there are also good and helpful lectins, e.g. in garlic, bitter gherkins and other Amara as well as wild herbs. They paralyze viruses and can destroy cancer cells.

However, the body also has natural mechanisms to keep lectins away. This includes, first of all, the *acidity of the stomach*, which, however, may be a deficiency of all people in blood group A from the outset, or in old age.

Furthermore, the continuous *mucus road* in the entire digestive tract helps. It is actively formed in the gut by certain bacteria (B. muciniphila Ackermansia, Faecali Prausnitzi), which is why a healthy *intestinal flora* is crucial for us. But not only for that, but because all vegetables must first pre-digested by our microflora, otherwise we could not absorb the ingredients. It also destroys many harmful lectins.

Glucosamina, a sugar-amino acid compound, binds lectins in the gut, which also increases tolerability. However, it must be added separately (for example, as Glukosa-K2®) because it is not included in the usual food. It has many more positive qualities, so it's worth the effort to supply.

Soya should only be eaten fermented, because it is containing phytates that impede many of the important nutrients in the intake, but not only that. They also inhibit trypsin and can cause extreme stress on the pancreas, which can promote cancer.

Also to be considered are origin and season. Only seasonal fruits and vegetables from the region should be used. However, this does not apply to milk and its products. These should be from southern Europe, because they contain the better-tolerated A2-beta-casein and not the incriminating A1-beta-casein. It can also trigger autoimmune reactions, including type I diabetes, because it attaches to the pancreatic beta cells responsible for insulin production.

The choice of nutrition depends not only on the type and appearance of the food selection, but on the freshness of a special kind. The good taste and the special value for health arises namely primarily by the content of *free electrons*. This can be determined by the so-called redox potential, which is actually investigated in some (unfortunately only a few) laboratories.

However, the content of electrons decreases increasingly, the longer the vegetables are stored after harvesting, or in the sun on the market stall. Shock-frozen vegetables, e.g. spinach are therefore clearly better, tastier and healthier! This is also related to the cold shock proteins that are formed.

Electrons play the decisive role in cell metabolism. But with every electric kitchen appliance, they are torn out of the fruit or vegetables and make it energetically worthless. Not only that: The lack of electrons makes healthy food (including juices) harmful radicals, i.e. electron robbers. Unfortunately that also applies to the so popular smoothies.

Additives in processed foods should always be viewed critically. Some of these are proven to be harmful to health. These include the preservative BHT (Butylhydroxytoluol), which may be listed under E 321. It is estrogen-like and is present in all artificial baked goods (biscuits, crackers, bars, etc.). There usually even cheaper corn syrup added for sweetening, with a high potential to create a fatty liver disease!

In addition, attention must be paid to artificial Trans-fats, which may appear as "emulsifiers" or as E 471, 472 and 475.

All plastic packaging and plastic bottles (including PET) contain plasticizers (phthalates) that block the thyroid hormone T_3 and thus the mitochondria. Not only because of this are they said to be involved in the development of cancer. However, the blockade of the T_3 receptor is not reflected in the blood levels!

Another problem is too much calcium in the diet, especially with the simultaneous consumption of phosphate. This is the case in concentrated form in processed cheese. According to Prof Makato Kuro-o, a well-known researcher of age is the consumption of calcium together with phosphate is suicide in instalments. Similar conditions are in fast food. Maxi stress is induced by Hamburger with processed cheese and Cola!
Phosphate is an antioxidant in many preservatives (acidulates!), Listed under E 339-341 and E 450-452 and also in flavour enhancers, H-milk, milk powder, kohlrabi (!) and especially baking soda and sausage – except in organic sausage!

When eating sea fish, make sure that almost all fish contain mercury. In the bigger ones, however, much more can be expected because of the longer life span than in the smaller ones. This should also be taken into account when taking fish oil as a dietary supplement. A good alternative is the high-quality *Neptune ™ Krill Oil NKO*, which is more expensive, but brings the greatest health benefits.

Warning is generally against over-strict, one-sided diets. This includes e.g. the vegan diet. It is not a healthy diet, as unfortunately is often taught, but a malnutrition that can cause significant health damage, especially in adolescent children, as brain development suffers.

However, as an introduction to a profound treatment of chronic illnesses, a comprehensive dietary change is indispensable. For at least 60%, in cancer even 80% of the disease development is attributable to a wrong, not type-appropriate diet.

Since in most cases an excess of easily digestible carbohydrates is responsible for this, it is recommended to start with the 6-week diet according to J. Schole, which, however, must be strictly followed. Strong bread eaters and cake friends need to be well motivated. But it's worth it!

Patients should strictly avoid for 6 weeks:
- ✖ any kind of potatoes
- ✖ rice
- ✖ corn
- ✖ cereals of all kinds, including chia, quinoa, etc.
- ✖ cooked root vegetables (including carrots!)
- ✖ sugar, honey, sweet fruits

Contraindications: Sarcoidosis, liver cirrhosis, seropositive rheumatism.

After just one week, a mostly unknown well-being effect occurs, clear thinking and good sleep. Often, these patients wish to carry on, which is possible, but is recommended only in a limited form, i.e. simply eating significantly less of the forbidden foods.
Burdens only arise when *too much and too often* food is eaten of the less recommended substances.

However, those who would love to eat cake or other carbohydrate bombs can do it! But they have to start walking tight after 30 minutes. Then the blood sugar does not rise and the growth hormone HGH is not blocked by insulin, which is the stated goal.

Some patients have a hard time getting a good breakfast on the Schole diet. This is a good reason – among many others – to fall back on the diet of Dr Johanna Budwig, with the linseed oil not only enough

Omega 3 oils are supplied, but above all (!) very many free electrons! This is not possible with any other food.

The recipe is:
- 125 g (organic) lean quark
- 3 – 5 big tablespoons fresh (!) linseed organic oil (depending on the size of the spoon)
- 3 – 5 tablespoons goat or sheep's milk
- 1 small tablespoon honey (not for diabetes or cancer)
- 2 big tablespoons of flaxseed (but only women)
- nuts or almonds

The mixture may only be mixed with a wooden spoon. Never use a mixer! Consume immediately after preparation.
Since the quality of the linseed oil is very important, a good oil mill should be selected (will be delivered) and should be ordered only small bottles.

This linseed-and-quark mixture can also be savoury with onions and spices. It replaces a whole meal.

Movement
The need is clear to most people, but often lacks implementation. This becomes a problem with the generally increasing obesity. Obesity is only the superficial symptom of a serious problem. Behind it is always a fatty liver (NAFLD), which is responsible for several diseases: diabetes, arteriosclerosis, heart attack, stroke...

Besides reducing carbohydrates, reducing food intake in the evening, and maintaining rhythms, it is good practice to walk around right after a meal and walk for at least 20 minutes (walking fast, such as Nordic walking). Although the optimum is 40 minutes / day, it can be reduced in time with strength training. These can also be pushups, squats or isometric exercises. Dumbbells are not necessary.

Attention: The higher the overweight, the more the movement should be in the direction of strength training to protect the joints!

Also be warned against exaggeration. Every effort requires a correspondingly long recovery period. The mentioned 40 minutes / day represent the optimum, but also the maximum! Anything beyond that takes more than 24 hours of convalescence. So if you want to exercise longer, you need at least one day break in between.

Sleep
Any regeneration can only take place in peace, what the night is for. In addition to the growth hormone, which is necessary for this, we need melatonin, which can be released only in complete darkness, but only if there exist no electro-smog. Cell phones or smartphones, computers, TVs and especially Wi-Fi belong not into the bedroom! The effects of these microwaves on our health are devastating. The research results are still kept under wraps. It is particularly critical with the expansion of the fast Internet to 5G standard. Any responsible citizen should inform themselves about this.
Without healthy sleep architecture with a variety of deep sleep and REM phases, no healing process can take place in an orderly fashion. That cannot be emphasized enough. This strengthens the kidneys, the quiescent pole for collective coherence, as a prerequisite for the high dynamics of cell metabolism.

Epilogue
Every cure is accompanied by a change of consciousness, otherwise it is only symptom elimination, and the disease would have had no meaning, just as everything in life has a higher meaning.

Spirit expresses itself in material reality, even in a source of illness. This shows a loss of order due to a lack of focus on the divinity of creation.

Matter consists of over a billion of interaction quanta ordered by information into fields and structure. The necessary energy comes from the same source – the light. Photons are the carriers of life information (from the sun) and are transported by electrons through the body. That is why electricity is the basic energy of the body. So does the cell metabolism as well as any power transmission.

Life can exist only if it constantly challenges itself. Construction goes hand in hand with dismantling. This ensures the constant renewal, but also creates problems when this balance is disturbed, e.g. in cancer.

Between the material components, relationships are built up that enable polar electrical voltages, as well as between the inner and outer cell milieu. To realize it, ATP must be provided. But only with good thyroid performance the required body temperature of 37 ° (98, 6° F) is reached. Already below 36.5°C is switched to glycolysis in the cytosol (fermentation).

The internal and external heat is therefore essential. In addition, communities are useful for facilitating an empathic encounter. It used to be survival. But even today creates the cohesion that transmits to all our cells and tissues. This is called collective coherence. It allows the high dynamics of all life processes, but requires a stable calm. This function is fulfilled by our kidneys. According to TCM, they are weakened by existential fears that reduce the basic trust in creation.

But everything is subject to a higher meaning: To gain experience through events that benefit the entire creation. Therefore, our existence is a service for a higher cause. For understanding this requires an expanded consciousness.

List of Figures

Figures page

1 Quantum physics describes interactions   9

2 The UNITED life supporting MEDICINE is not only holistically oriented, but fully considers the interactions of all systems with each other. In this case, the superordinate control of matter by the spirit is given the due importance.   12

3 Using the example of the 4 sex hormones, the bi-polar conditions can be displayed very well. Progesterone is the antagonist of the oestrogens and cortisol the antagonist of the testosterone. Each axle strives for a dynamic balance and thus low energy consumption.   14

4 This selection shows the hierarchy of functional systems from the centre outwards. Changes in a quadrant, e.g. blue's *self-satisfaction* will first affect the overlying cell metabolism and underlying acids-base homeostasis and then gradually spread to the blue quadrants of all other planes.   16

5 The bipolar regulation of cell metabolism. Anabolic peptides can replace HGH, which can be blocked by insulin as well as permanent psychic stress. However, if these remain elevated after an acute illness   17

for a longer period of time, chronification occurs because the cortisol receptors on the nucleus are already degraded on the 8th day.

6 The regulation of cell metabolism in the usual four- pole representation. It should be noted that the (yellow-green) separation axis is controlled by the *reciprocally* arranged integration axis and vice versa. Disturbances on one of these polar axes therefore have their cause on the other. At the edge the meaning of the quadrants for the organism is listed. In particular, the temperature-dependent mode of energy generation plays a major role. The lower limit for normal mitochondrial function is 36,5 ° C (97,7° F). 19

7 The Luescher cube and the 4 self-esteems. Only when all 4 are realized can we live in *harmony*. Harmony is the balance of all polar opposites. 23

8 All diseases can be assigned to the 4 quadrants. This not only makes it easier to identify the cause, but also to derive a deeply effective therapy from it. 26

9 Interactions of the organ systems 26

10 Generation of the healing information in the frontal brain of the patients by mirror neurons. 29

11 Monitor image of the 4-pole regulation of cell 32

metabolism in conjunction with the acids-base balance. The 4 Luescher colours refer to the higher positioned psycho regulation. You can see the ground state, where all 4 colour points are on the inner circle. For the assessment, however, it is not a normal "state" that is crucial, but the dynamics in the adaptation to changing environmental influences, which is reflected in the movement around the middle position.

12 The therapy principle of the 4 quadrants according to the rules of TCM (5 conversion phases). With bioelectronic devices such as the ZMR 703 and the diagnostic module of the MORA*nova*, a treatment can be fully automatic.   38

13 The principle of polar equalization can be understood very well in this illustration. No matter on which level – integration and separation axes always have to be balanced.   39

14 Since reality is fundamentally switched via emotions, the transformation of stressful situations and emotions stored (!) in the interference field is a *conditio sine qua non* for the healing process. In addition to the MRT 503 and the NEC 708 headphones, a special cable set is required to perform the treatment.   42

15 Diet chart   48

Literature

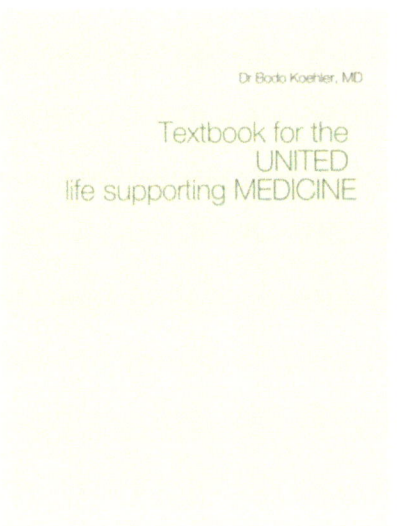

The textbook of the UNITED life supporting MEDICINE sets new standards in the diagnosis and treatment of chronically ill patients. It has translated the research results of eminent scientists into practice and thus points the way for a long overdue union of conventional medicine and naturopathy. This step leads to another dimension of medicine, through the integration of synergistic methods. This results in a new quality, with which the long overdue paradigm shift can be initiated. To this end, quantum physics has contributed significantly and opened up new perspectives.

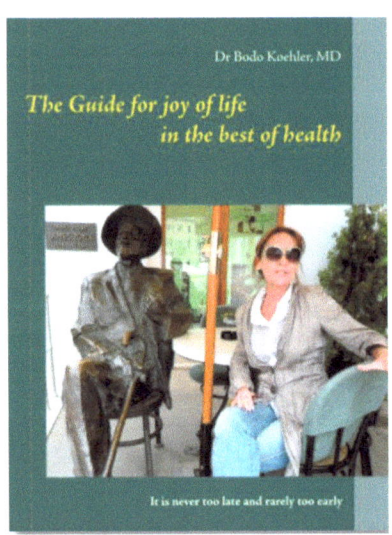

The Guide for joy deals with important everyday issues, starting with nutrition, lifestyle, philosophical issues of life and medical problems, especially if they are caused by the widespread errors of medicine. It is the concern of the author to address and clear up them openly, e.g. about civilization disorders such as arteriosclerosis, osteoporosis, etc. This book provides extensive experience gained in over 45 years of professional activity as an internist and naturopathic physician. There is often a contrary view of the prevailing opinion in the room, but which can be scientifically justified.

Living Systems Information Therapy – Introduction to Quantum Medicine; Volume I and II, Textbook for the doctor and naturopath practice, 1th edition in English 2019

This fundamental work describes the physical connections behind the phenomena of our reality. Living Systems Information Therapy LSIT is able to initiate healing processes even in advanced chronic diseases.

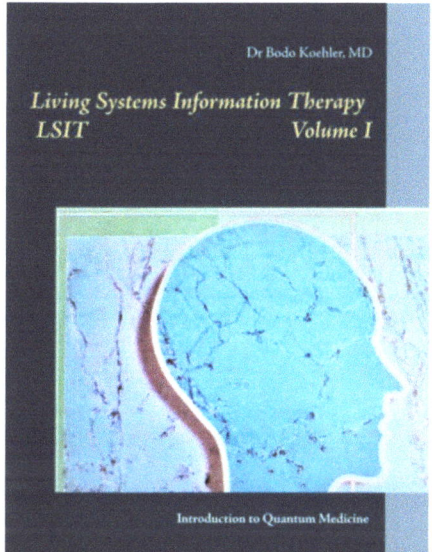
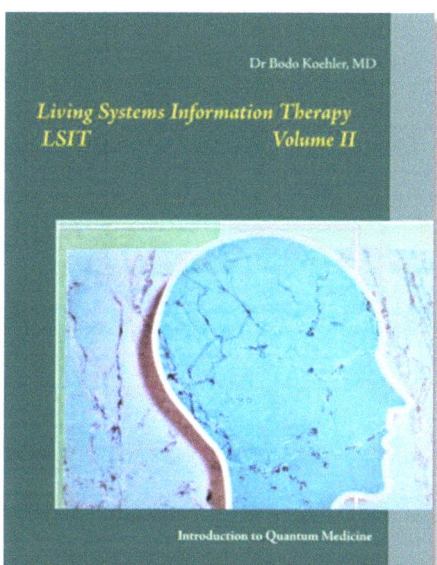

In some indications, for example allergies, intoxications and the like, it is unsurpassed.

The textbook comprehensively and understandable discusses the physical and biomedical foundations of Living Systems Information Therapy LSIT with internal and external signals, and the "how to do" approach to success-fully apply this more and more adherent therapy to the benefit of the patient.

Attachment

In order to be able to put the theory into practice safely, a few principles must be observed:
Even if usually only a specific area of the body is affected, this is affecting the *whole organism*. The cohesion, which can also be called coherence, is lost.

However, it can also be stated in reverse: All individual problems of a person are projected onto the *weakest point* and manifest themselves there as a symptom. There are therefore always several causes, ranging from malnutrition, microbes, heavy metals and to mental stress – which can overwhelm the system "man" as a whole. Therefore, the view of the whole should never be obscured by individual findings.

4 aspects of body organization

The four main areas concern (see Fig. I):
- ➢ The ability to find inner peace and good sleep quality
- ➢ The functionality of the microflora, inside and out
- ➢ The synthesis and detoxification function of the liver
- ➢ Energy production at normal body temperature.

Nothing works without energy, but without a sufficiently high body temperature of at least 36.5 ° C (97, 7 ° F core temperature); there is no ATP production in the mitochondria. Then only glycolysis in the cytosol takes place, producing only $1/19^{th}$ of ATP.
An essential condition for health (and every healing process!) is therefore a normal thyroid function. However, if thyroxine in the liver cannot be cleaved to T_3, or if receptor blockages are present (for example, by WGA), the body does not get up to speed either.

Meanwhile, the liver is in the foreground when it comes to the "usual" civilization diseases such as diabetes, arteriosclerosis or even cancer. Unfortunately, a badly to diagnose fatty liver NAFLD significantly impedes liver metabolism, which has serious effects on the whole organism. Only by consistent carbohydrate restriction, including the fructose (!), the fat in the liver can be broken down. This also includes adjusted movement (overweight people should prefer strength training), possibly also short-term fasting, and the associated insulin resistance may disappear again.

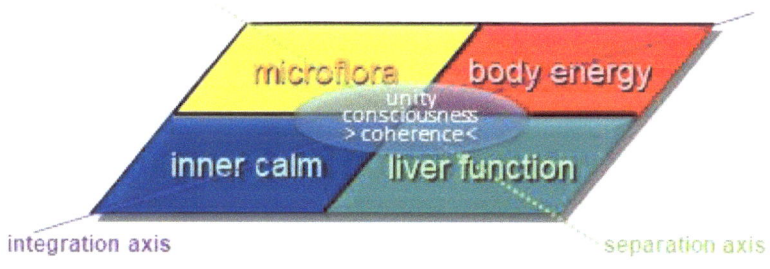

© Dr Bodo Koehler, MD

Fig. I: All 4 aspects belong together and should not be considered in isolation. Only in an optimally balanced situation can high coherence be achieved as a prerequisite for health.

The intestinal flora also has a strong effect on the liver, as it produces important metabolites, especially for the immune system, under natural conditions (acidic pH!) and the right composition (Fig. II). In an alkaline environment, putrefaction bacteria that produce harmful ammonia nest. Therefore, always ensure sufficient acidity in the diet and avoid acid blockers in any case! The older a person, the more must be expected with a gastric acid deficiency, with all the negative consequences (B12 deficiency, anaemia, etc.).

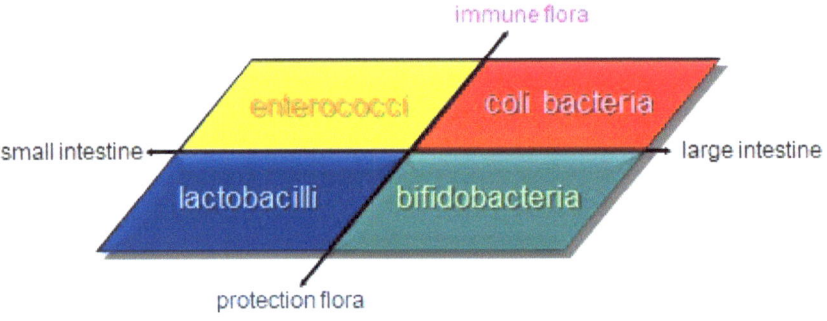

Fig. II: It depends on these four main tribes. They should be sufficiently present and find their physiological acidic environment in the intestine.

The biggest carriers of microbes are in descending order intestines, lungs, skin and brain! There are mainly viruses located, but they interact with the gut via the vagus nerve. This means that the more optimal the intestinal flora is put together, the lower the virulence of the viruses that can infect the brain! This is especially important in neuro-degenerative diseases such as Parkinson's, Alzheimer's etc.

The microbiome creates the basis for the function of the *immune system*. Due to the ever-changing environmental conditions, especially by **electro-smog**, the loads are constantly increasing, which requires increased combat readiness. At the same time, however, tolerance must be practiced. Intensive training is required for this tightrope walk, for which in addition to the thymus is responsible for our intestinal flora, as it is the first stop on the way into the body. A weak immune reaction as well as an excessive (allergic) indicates a disturbed composition of the flora.

The following steps have proved successful:
- Stool diagnostics in the special laboratory
- Colon cleansing (10 days, rinses, enemas) KlinSiMag®!
- Tolerance increasing (coli bacteri + enterococchi)
- Immune flora > enterococchi and coli
- Protective flora (bifid bacteria, lactobacilli) = settling flora
- Milieu boost (vinegar, lemon, lactic acid) pH 5.8-6.5!
- "Feed" (inulin, glutamic acid, brewer's yeast)
- Liver support (Silymarin, Amara = CurSiMag®)
- Attention leaky gut! (colostrum, Krill Oil, KlinSiMag®)

The most important aspect in Fig. I is the blue quadrant. Today we live in a hurried society that is striving for more and more growth and has completely supplanted the very cause of existence.

We are spiritual beings and derive our entire existence from the non-material universe. Quantum physicists use different terms such as zero-point field, vacuum, quantum space, etc., or simply SPIRIT. From "there" we get our life information, which is sent to us through the sun in the form of coded photons.

Also from this source comes the information that enriches and makes us happy. However, it is necessary to have meditative contact with our origin. This should be done automatically at night; otherwise all the atheists would have died long ago. But we can also actively establish contact by going into the "quantum mechanical ground state". Only then is healing or health possible.

However, the blue quadrant is much more comprehensive. He shows our relationship skills. Relationships should serve to achieve something together that would not be possible on their own. That's the potential we should use. Because at the same time we become more resilient, because a good relationship creates trust and thus reduces fears. Then we can rest in ourselves, even if the world collapses around us.

Only when all 4 aspects of health have been optimized can appear the unified state, which we call coherence. But this is not a passive act, but a state of consciousness, which we should active strive for.
Everything can communicate again undisturbed with everything, every information is reachable everywhere, what we call quantum state. And that is nothing else but universal LOVE.

Application of the categorical order system

The *categorical order system*, which unites all functional systems, can also be very useful in everyday life. So here are a few hints for the right application.

First, that system should be clearly defined, which should be put into a categorical order. It must always be a self-contained functional unit whose components are in direct interaction with each other. The example of a *family* is easy to understand. It is undoubtedly clear who belongs to it and who does not. Generally these are the following 4 components: mother (blue), father (red), child(ren) (green) and grandparents (yellow). These communicate with each other, but also with other families, on the same (experience) level because of similar experience content that can be exchanged. This provides easy access to these similarities.

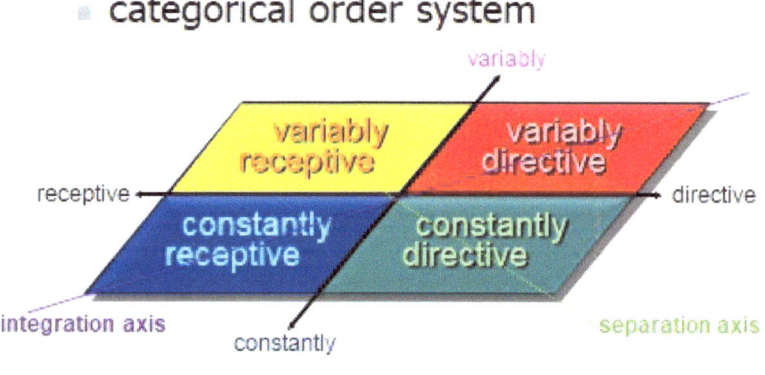

Fig. III: The Luescher cube is indispensable for correct scientific work. In this figure, only the middle floor is shown.

This principle can be extended and applied upwards (community, state) and downwards (cells, structures). Because of its special importance, we take the cell metabolism as an example here.

The cell metabolism is (according to J. Schole) regulated by 4 components: HGH – the growth hormone, thyroxine, the thyroid hormone and cortisol, an important stress hormone and anti-inflammatory substance. We have to add the anabolic peptides, which can be responsible for a prolonged inflammation.

For the correct assignment, the following decisions should be made successively:

1. Is the component to be judged directive or receptive? HGH is certainly receptive because it is secreted on demand by the pituitary gland, e.g. at each cell division, since it is responsible for differentiation and maturation.

2. Is the component variable or constant? HGH remains constant in the blood if it is not blocked by insulin or prolonged psychic stress. Thus HGH belongs in the blue quadrant.

3. Now follows a review. Is HGH integrative or separative? It is, of course, integrative, because it supports the maintenance of the cell state. And: Does it correspond to the properties of the water element? Yes, definitely. It reinforces the coherence.

Thus, the assignment is correct into the ***blue quadrant***.

Applying this scheme to the other 3 components, we can see, that thyroxine combines all the properties of the red quadrant: variably-directive, integrative, and possesses the properties of the fire element, the maintenance of body heat.

For cortisol (yellow) and the anabolic peptides (green) the assignment is only a matter of form. The correct overall result can be seen in Fig. 6 on page 19.

A functional system always includes 4 similar components, two of which face each other polar. This can be done a further review of the assignment. On the axis of integration this is true for HGH and thyroxine as well as on the separation axis for cortisol (anti-inflammatory drug) and anabolic peptides (inflammatory adjuvants). Thus, the categorical classification for the 4-pole regulated cell metabolism was successful, and this principle can now be applied to other systems.

Load capacity of the organism
Turning now to Fig. IV, we can present the resilience of the organism, its strengths and weaknesses, quite individually.

The lifestyle settles here and influences the system. This includes good or bad nutrition, which also has a direct effect on the microbiome. Not negligible is the psychic aspect. Fear of the future, fear of life, lack of fulfilment – all this concerns the yellow quadrant.

At the same time the liver at the opposite pol can suffer as a result. In other words, in yellow is a good way to strengthen (or weaken) the liver. Thus we have grasped the separation axis and thus an overview of the (homemade) predisposition.

The axis of integration now decides how well or how bad the influence from outside affects. In the blue sits the relationship ability and thus the opportunity to get new information or to plan joint projects. Here is the *sensation* at home, positive or negative, with which we control the reality. This generates emotions that are translated into the red quadrant.

Existential fears in the blue or lack of will due to lack of self-confidence (- - red) prevent this.

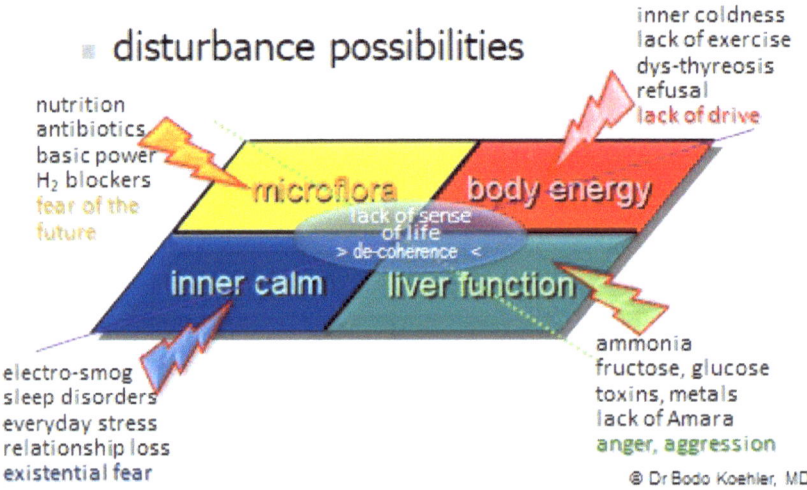

Fig. IV: All types of interference possibilities should be taken into account. Health can be achieved by largely eliminating these influences, but also by increasing the resistance. However, none of the 4 aspects must be missing.

Consequences

Basically, for thinking in the UNITED MEDICINE:

Less is more! Regulatory ability is everything!

In concrete terms, everything should be eliminated first, which could be a factor of interfering, before we apply any medication. The regulation is always blocked by a too much, no matter at what level. In addition, the environment is always in the first place.

Yellow is about the relationship to the environment and personal environment. This includes the inside of the intestine and the lungs, as it still belongs to the outside world. The necessary, constant regeneration of the contact surfaces is dependent on stable, acidic conditions. These must be taken care of first. This not only affects the mucous membranes, but also the skin itself.

In green, structure and order play the main role. Harmful substances should be removed from the diet. This includes fast food. However, more and more important is the recognition and relieving of a fatty liver, a problem of our time.

The integration axis blue-red should be considered as a whole in terms of its ability to be regulated, since the function of the separation axis depends on this. Every person should therefore generate his personal haven of peace, to which he can always find his way back, especially in difficult situations, be it through autogenic training (AT), meditation or turning to GOD. Only in calm is the strength for all necessary actions, but also for recovery.

In order for the necessary energy to be provided in red, the mitochondria need to be functional. This is only possible with a core temperature above 36.5 ° C (97,7 ° F). Therefore, enough thyroxine must be present. That should be guaranteed. Then it is easier to implement a personal exercise program.

If these 4 points are consistently implemented, the necessary healing requirements are available on a physical level. However, that does not help anything if life is not geared towards a purpose that is implemented with joy and love. Only then can the necessary coherence be achieved.

List of Figures 2

Figures   **page**

I   All 4 aspects belong together and should not be considered in isolation. Only in an optimally balanced situation can high coherence be achieved as a prerequisite for health.   63

II   It depends on these four main tribes. They should be sufficiently present and find their physiological acidic environment in the intestine.   64

III   The Luescher cube is indispensable for correct scientific work. In this figure, only the middle floor is shown   67

IV   All types of interference possibilities should be taken into account. Health can be achieved by largely eliminating these influences, but also by increasing the resistance. However, none of the 4 aspects must be missing   70

Curious? Would like more? Then you are ready for the textbook of the UNITED MEDICINE! I wish you success!

XXX